JUST HEAL, BRO.
JOURNAL

JAY BARNETT

Just HEAL Bro. Journal
©2021 by Jay Barnett
ISBN: 978-0-578-96687-8

Cover by Jared Michael Design Co.
Text design by Lisa DeSpain, www.book2bestseller.com

CONTENTS

Dealing with the Future

ACKNOWLEDGEMENTS

I give all praise to God for choosing me as a vessel to help many take the journey of healing, and I'm forever grateful to be a voice and instrument.

Also, I want to thank my family for always supporting my purpose to help others grow and evolve beyond their experiences.

Most importantly, I'm grateful for my tribe of brothers: thank you to Greg, Spence, Shawn, Alfred, Bishop Borders, Big G (Garrick), Rob, Hassan, Seto, Tony Jones, Lincoln, Prophet Hector, and Shareeff.

You guys created space for me when I was at my lowest, and I was inspired by each of you to create this journal to promote a brotherhood of men from all walks of life.

Thank you.

FOREWORD

"And the Lord said, Simon, Simon, behold, Satan hath desired to have you, that he may sift you as wheat: But I have prayed for thee, that thy faith fail not: and when thou art converted, strengthen thy brethren."

—Luke 22:31-32 KJV

It's the "when thou art converted" for me, bro. That was the hardest part. The conversion. The conversion of sadness, loneliness, depression, self-medication, self-doubt, and fornication (likely because of how little I valued myself). While I was healing from divorce, I was raising my son in the house I had been married in and sleeping in the same bed where we had conceived my miracle son. That was the fight of my life.

As I reflect on my journey, I recall the many men I talked to along the way who were experiencing some of the same things I'd experienced in life: abuse, child custody negotiations, divorce settlements, and balancing being a high achiever when you are at heart a homebody. Add being a Black man born in Texas (which is the South and its own country at the same time), sometimes I felt like an alien. I still do and probably always will.

Being an alien, feeling like I was the only one going through what I was going through, didn't always mean I was alienated. I found a common thread and theme amongst us men. We simply have few places that are "safe." No, not the barbershop. No, not the locker room. No, not the golf course. And sometimes not even the men's ministry at church. Where can we keep it real? For me, the first place to start was to find a safe place *for* myself and *in* myself. I needed a place where I could be honest and vulnerable, while trying to forgive myself. As I started to let go of the shame I felt for all the situations that had been unfolding as my "star" was rising, I found myself at the intersection of choosing life or death.

The one thing we need most is healing, the necessary conversion when the devil tries to "sift you." Sifting is when the devil has desired you, and you fell into his trap. Wait—does the devil have a gender pronoun? We could use a few other adjectives and pronouns to describe the enemy, but what we call the devil isn't that important. The important thing is to recognize how God dealt with the enemy on your behalf on your road to healing and the boundaries you place around this known enemy. God will deal with your enemy and provide you with wisdom, knowledge, love, and joy to you along your path. Be sure to record this or at least remember it, because WHAT YOU ARE GOING THROUGH ISN'T REALLY FOR YOU.

Habakkuk 2:2 says, "And the Lord answered me, and said, Write the vision, and make it plain upon tables, that he may run that readeth it." In other words, God told the prophet Habakkuk to record the vision of what he saw for getting out of a potential disaster. A chapter before that, Habbakuk is characterized as being burdened by sight: "The burden which Habakkuk the prophet did see" Habakkuk 1:1.

Brother, are you burdened with something you've seen, experienced, or been traumatized by? If so, write it down. Write down the things you haven't told your family, your spouse, your closest friends, and perhaps even yourself. But don't just write about the past. Cast your vision for your future, regardless of your past or current failures and tragedies. Spend some time recording the vision lying deep within your soul. This journal will be a life raft for you.

If someone happens to find your writings, they might be a healing salve or catalytic converter for them. Someone needs to hear your story and how you overcame your circumstances. They need to know how you became who you are, despite the devil trying to remind you of who you used to be. This shared journey is iron sharpening iron, strengthening your brothers and sisters.

My hope for you, my brother, is that you dig deep, write through your tears, and celebrate in your triumphs. You are triumphant. You are a king. You are worthy. You are enough. And you are healed, even if you don't feel it. You are healed. If you are fighting your belief in these things, "Just Do It," like Nike says, but even better—Just Heal, Bro!

—Lincoln Stephens

DEALING WITH THE PAST

MY BROTHER,

It is with great honor and humility that I greet you. My healing journey has been just that, a journey that began ten years ago after my second suicide attempt. I decided if God allowed me another opportunity to live, then I must have a PURPOSE.

Purpose is the *reason* something is done or created. I discovered this meaning as I begin to grow and heal from my childhood pains and traumas. We all have purpose, but sometimes life happens, and we are blinded by circumstances and situations that occur and cause us to believe otherwise.

My mission with this journal is for you to begin the healing process as you write your thoughts. As men, it is challenging for us to open up because many of us didn't have safe spaces when we were boys to be emotionally vulnerable.

I want this journal to be *your* safe place, brother. You can no longer wait on someone else to provide safety for you. You must first become safe for yourself. As you take this journey, be intentional as often as you can as you sit with yourself. Reflect and process and be introspective. Take a deep look within and begin to rebuild and repair as you record your thoughts.

Journaling is a tool. It can improve your self-awareness and promote positive thinking. It can also help declutter the fogginess of your brain that can cause anxiety and depression. When you sit down to write, lean into the moment, and feel everything during that time. Feel the pain of your past, allow your feelings to roam, and let your thoughts flow.

This is your time, brother, and you deserve to live a HEALED LIFE.

I hope this journal helps to bring clarity and insight like never before, and you begin to THRIVE rather than just survive.

Just Heal, Bro

—King Jay

WHAT HAPPENED?

Many times, who you are or who you think you are has been shaped by your experiences. Today I want you to take a journey of some life encounters that may have created a persona or maladaptive behaviors.

Maladaptive behaviors (behaviors that stop you from adapting to new or difficult circumstances) usually start after a traumatic event or major life change. For many people, they picked up these habits at an early age.

What was a major event in your life that changed you?

_____

_____

_____

_____

_____

_____

_____

How old were you when it happened?

_____

_____

_____

_____

_____

_____

_____

_____

What habits or behaviors did you adopt after the event?

_____

_____

_____

_____

_____

_____

_____

_____

_____

_____

Write down what you are feeling as you recall the event or experience.

_____

_____

_____

_____

_____

_____

_____

_____

Write down 5 things you have learned about yourself during the process of journaling about it.

_____

_____

_____

_____

_____

_____

_____

_____

Remember, "YOU ARE NOT what happened to you." Take back your power by releasing the narrative that you are the experience. You are healing, brother, and life is adjusting to your healed mindset.

FORGIVENESS FOR WHAT?

Forgiveness and healing go hand in hand; you cannot have one without the other. Forgiveness is an action and it's never easy, bro. It can be one of the hardest things you do in life, especially when the people who hurt you will never apologize.

Your healing is on the other side of forgiveness. Don't carry bitterness and resentment throughout life. That is dangerous, my brother.

I spent most of my life hating my father because of what he did to my mother. He abandoned me when they divorced. Later when I played ball, I would envision my dad's face on my opponent, and I would try to destroy them because I wanted revenge. But as I went through life, the anger affected my quality of living, and my unforgiveness wouldn't let me receive love or give it properly.

Forgiveness is hard, bro, but it's necessary if you want to live a life of freedom. Take time this week to really feel everything you have been holding in toward anyone who has wronged you.

"Forgiveness is for YOU, not for them."

Who is the person you feel unforgiveness toward?

_____

_____

_____

_____

_____

_____

_____

_____

What did they do? (Let's talk about it.)

_____

_____

_____

_____

_____

_____

_____

_____

_____

Have you forgiven yourself?

_____

_____

_____

_____

_____

_____

_____

_____

Describe your pain in detail.

_____

_____

_____

_____

_____

_____

_____

_____

_____

_____

_____

Forgiveness gives us the power to live beyond the event or experience that once held us captive. When we hold on to the pain and choose not to forgive, we give up our power to the one who wounded us. This causes fear in us because we give them power to control every aspect of our life.

How would forgiving that person free you?

Write a letter to the individual who caused the pain you're feeling. Release as much of your feelings as you can. When you're done, tear the page up into tiny pieces and BURN them.

WHAT IF?

The world tells you I am hard, tough, and emotionless, but what if you discovered I was the complete opposite?

Actually, I am softer than you think. While I'm stern and solid when I need to be, my hard exterior is just a defense mechanism to block outsiders who pretend they care about me. I have emotions too, believe it or not. I have feelings about many different things, but I find it difficult to share them. I am not sure what would happen if I shared them.

Many times, I have wanted to cry, but I didn't feel I could. I had all these expectations to hold it together, and I had to be stoic and stand tall when I really wanted to fall apart.

The same world that told you I was hard, tough, and emotionless never provided space for me to just be. To be even more transparent, the same world will take my athletic ability and put it on center stage but will shoot me if I don't comply with their standards or rules.

They just said, "Be a Man," but what does that mean to a boy who has never seen a man? Most of the men I saw didn't cry or show emotion. As a matter of fact, they acted as if they didn't care. That is what I have been doing, but I am tired of acting like a machine. I want to feel, I want to be heard, and I want to be seen as a human being, not just for what I can provide.

What if?

What if everything the world told you about me was completely wrong? What would you do?

Would you exploit my insecurities? Would you tell everyone I shared my deepest secrets with you, and now you're questioning my masculinity? How would you have handled me being sexually abused, knowing that now I hide behind sex to cover up the pain? Would you emotionally blackmail me because I failed to meet your expectations of a man?

Most men have been taught that a woman's needs are more important, and our only concerns should be providing and protecting. I believe wholeheartedly that our needs are equally important, even though they're different in context.

Can I be honest?

I really want to fall apart and show you I am none of the things society has told you about me. I am scared most of the time, but I'm afraid to tell you because I'm not sure how you would see me. I want to tell you that some bad things happened to me when I was a kid too, but will you question my sexuality? There have been many times I wanted to open my heart for love, but I have never seen a healthy relationship or what a real man looks like.

What if you could see that I was winging this whole "man" thing?

Would you say I am weak and can do nothing for you because I'm soft and too emotional as a man? The truth of the matter is I am neither soft nor too emotional; I am HUMAN, just like you.

I just want to feel safe and know what I share won't be weaponized against me. I want to know that you won't keep score of my shortcomings and will provide a safe space for me. The same world we live in doesn't accept me either way. Daily I smile and wear a cape full of holes while I pretend I am Superman.

I really want to show them I am Clark Kent. There is no phone booth for me to change in; I just want to be.

What if?

What if you listened to me to understand me? Sometimes I don't know how to put my words together like you. Sometimes my words come in waves, but that's my way of processing, not me deflecting.

What if we both could just feel without reservations and be compassionate without judging or criticizing?

As men and women, we're similar in many ways yet different in how we express ourselves, according to our function, and that's ok. It's the way God made us so we can work together. It would be redundant for us both to have the same level of function. That would make us the same.

Brothers want to feel safe as well. We just need safe spaces to be and not fear that we will be exploited.

What if?

What if you saw the little boy I am protecting from being hurt? Would you provide safety for the man who is hiding behind him?

This piece is dedicated to all the brothers who are seeking safety from someone they love.

—King Jay

DEALING WITH THE PRESENT

THOUGHTS OF INADEQUACY

The feeling of not being enough is very common among men because we live in a world that judges us by our abilities rather than our character. Trust me, bro, it took a long time for me to believe in myself, and it was not easy.

Let's explore where your thoughts of inadequacy began so you can tear down the walls of false narratives.

What are your thoughts about yourself? Are they positive or negative?

_____

_____

_____

_____

_____

_____

_____

_____

Who or what shaped your thoughts about yourself?

_____

_____

_____

_____

_____

_____

_____

_____

Do any of the thoughts you have about yourself hold any truth as to who you really are? (Sit with this question before writing.)

_____

_____

_____

_____

_____

_____

_____

_____

_____

_____

Write five things you are adequate in (or really good at) and reestablish your OWN thoughts.

_____

_____

_____

_____

_____

_____

_____

_____

Create an affirmation that speaks against inadequate thoughts. Example: "I learn quickly and easily, and have fun with new information."

_____

_____

_____

_____

_____

_____

_____

_____

"Thoughts will come and go but you determine which thoughts will hold residence in your mind."

—King Jay

GOT BOUNDARIES?

Boundaries are essential for having a healthy relationship with yourself and others. Setting boundaries and sustaining them is a skill you must develop. Most men have never established their own boundaries, because they were taught to respect them in others but not have them for themselves. Take the time this week to identify your boundaries.

Boundaries are not for keeping people out; they're important for your own functioning to keep you centered within yourself. Take all the time you need, bro. Set your boundaries and stand on them.

What are some areas you have neglected that need some boundaries?

_____

_____

_____

_____

_____

_____

_____

What are your limits? You can't set good boundaries until you are clear about them, so identify your physical, emotional, mental, and spiritual boundaries.

_____

_____

_____

_____

_____

_____

_____

_____

Make YOU a priority. It's ok to give yourself permission to take care of yourself first; it's an act of self-respect and kindness toward you, bro.

Write down how you will begin to prioritize your own needs moving forward.

_____

_____

_____

_____

_____

_____

_____

Start small, bro. Just like getting better in sports, it will take repetition. Remember when coach said, "Get them reps in, guys." Do the same when you set your boundaries. Practice, practice, practice.

Write down how you will start setting boundaries.

_____

_____

_____

_____

_____

_____

_____

_____

_____

_____

_____

_____

_____

_____

_____

_____

_____

"Setting boundaries is an act of self-love. Don't stop loving yourself for nothing and no one because it's your responsibility."

—King Jay

VIOLATED

Cast out by those who said they loved me but often treated me like a black sheep, I fell in love with the wolves. Withdrawn from my reality, I created a persona to hide my truth. Living a lie felt easy until it became too hard to reveal my truth.

Smile on my face with an angry heart because it feels like being dead is better than being alive. Closing my curtains puts my anxiety at ease; turning off the lights drowns my pain. I'm so tired of this feeling like this, all day every day. Pill after pill, and my anxiety feels like it's getting worse. It's hard to sleep because my thoughts are still awake, and they want to talk to my dreams. My brain has extended conversations about how they won't miss me if I am gone. In a house full of people, I feel alone.

Yeah, I stunt on the gram. Who doesn't? I wouldn't dare let any of my followers know who I really am. For what? I will do what my parents do best: put on a facade like everything is perfect. After all, everyone life's is perfect on social media.

I'm not popular, but I'm well known for my dark and gloomy look. School feels like jail, and I'm a prisoner who is waiting for the warden to say, "Open cell block for inmate #285286." I just want to be free. I want to run far away from the injury that caused this confused state. They say I should see a therapist, but for what? Only for them to tell me I'm worse than I already know? I will just say what Mom and Dad want to hear: "I'm good bruh. Just give me my meds and let me be."

Another day. *Damn, I'm still here.* I was hoping someone would accidentally hit our car on the drive home. Put me out of my misery. That would be ideal because the reality is my family is fake. They say whatever it takes to appear perfect for their peers, while I hold on tight to these shears.

We haven't been to church in a while. Maybe that will help. Sunday morning comes, and I'm ready to show them the pastor can't fix what he didn't break. Holding onto my bible like it's my last breath, I would rather leave it at home because it's just a book to me. I'm dragged to the altar only to walk away, shining like a piece of silver from the oil on my forehead, glistening like the old man's Rolex. Imagine that: the blessed oil didn't help me either. I guess the miracle wasn't paid for, so I wasn't feeling any better. Only it's worse because my parents are imposters. Behind closed doors, the Jones's picture is taped on the refrigerator, and they still can't keep up.

Sitting in the back seat, I let my thoughts run into the depths of my mind. Daydreams are for planning, scene one, and action:

The door opens, Mom calls my name, and I don't answer. She walks around and begins screaming and crying hysterically. "My baby... whyyy??? Why???" She talks more than I ever heard her talk before. No note, just a response to the nonstop questions I never wanted to answer. This is what is wrong.

I'm suicidal. One shot to the right side of my head, pulled by my dominant hand. Dad runs up the stairs to comfort Mom. Just as I knew, he was emotionally unavailable. Instead of reaching down and asking his son, *why*, he just stands there. He was the same old money-chasing prick he's always been.

I played this scene out in my head on the ride home from church.
"Jared, Jared..."
"What, Mom?"
"We're home. Are you okay???"
"Yessss I'm good." Damn that felt real, and I'm tired of daydreaming. I'm ready to close out my reality for the actuality that I will no longer be here.

Oh yeah, you are probably wondering why I feel this pain. At the age of nine, the deacon of the church picked me up one day and said we were going to hang out. Mom and Dad told me to go have fun. Little did they know, the fun would come courtesy of the deacon's demons. We stopped for ice cream, and he said he was the cone and he wanted me to lick the ice cream off him. Confused and traumatized is the only way to describe how I felt that day. Yes, I was sexually abused and molested by the most trusted deacon of the church, according to my parents.

What am I supposed to do with this pain? Five years later and I'm the bad guy because I'm acting out of hurt that I can't let go of. The only way to eradicate this is to let go; I just want to DIE. I'm suicidal because I want to end the pain of the memory because I still have to see this monster roaming the church while I'm buried in the pain of the experience.

I'm stuck in this identity crisis. I'm struggling with who I want to become because the trauma has crippled my perception of myself. I don't know if I'm gay or straight. I didn't ask to be molested by someone who was supposed to be trusted. Now I'm sharing my truth of what happened to me on that day that changed my entire perspective on life.

When you judge me, my actions, and why I'm suicidal, don't ask, "Are you good?" Ask what HAPPENED??!

—King Jay

According to a review of child sex abuse prevalence studies, 1 in 25 boys will be sexually abused before they turn 18.

Most males may never report being victims of sexual abuse because of the stereotypes that exist in our culture pertaining to how males are supposed to be strong and independent. Society has done a huge disservice to our boys by pushing toxic messages that tell boys not to cry, and to instead man up.

I wrote this piece to help the brother who has experienced sexual abuse to feel comfortable sharing their story and truth.

WEAK POINTS

A mentor of mine, Bishop Randy Borders, once told me, "If you work in your strength, you stay in control of your weaknesses."

Honestly, I had to sit with this. I began to focus on the areas I was strong in rather than my weaknesses. I thought to myself, *this is some reverse psychology because I need to identify my weak spots.* However, as I locked in on my strengths, I quickly identified the areas that needed improvement.

We all have areas we can improve. It's critical to identify your weaknesses as soon as you can to identify your strong points.

For example, I'm consistent in most things I do, but one of my weaknesses was procrastination. What I realized is that when I focused on remaining consistent, I procrastinated less, and I was more productive. Bishop was right. The more I focused on my strengths, I maintained control of my weaknesses.

We are not Superman; we cannot leap tall buildings in a single bound, nor do we have a bat cave where Alfred is waiting to aid us in our conquests to save Gotham. Our weakness are very much real; however, we don't have to be consumed by them to improve and correct them.

Take the journey of identifying your weaknesses while exploring your areas of strength. List some areas where you are struggling to remain consistent and where you are limiting your success.

_____

_____

_____

_____

_____

_____

_____

_____

What does it mean to be weak? How has your weakness impacted your life?

_____

_____

_____

_____

_____

_____

_____

_____

How can you do a better job of working in your strong areas to combat your weak areas?

_____

_____

_____

_____

_____

_____

_____

_____

Create an affirmation for areas of improvement and remaining consistent in the things you do well.

_____

_____

_____

_____

_____

_____

_____

_____

"Focus on your strengths, not your weaknesses.
Focus on your character, not your reputation.
Focus on your blessings, not your misfortunes."
—Roy T. Bennett, *The Light in the Heart*

STRESSED

Stress is a silent killer that has conquered many men because they are unable to manage their levels of stress. By the time they recognize they're stressed, it's usually too late.

Stress affects men differently than women because men are more likely to have a fight or flight response.

How you respond to stress determines your outcome, so it's imperative you have the right skills to identify, manage, and control your stress levels and response. Believe it or not, stress causes many diseases. A U.S. national study reported that 60 to 80 percent of doctors' visits may include a stress-related component.

What have you been stressing about and how can you become better at reducing your stress?

_____

_____

_____

_____

_____

_____

What seems to stress you the most? Why?

_____

_____

_____

_____

_____

_____

_____

_____

How physically active are you when you're stressed? If you're not, explore the reasons why.

_____

_____

_____

_____

_____

_____

_____

_____

_____

How do the things that are out of your control stress you?

_____

_____

_____

_____

_____

_____

_____

_____

_____

What have you done in the past to manage your stress? Was it healthy?

_____

_____

_____

_____

_____

_____

_____

_____

_____

Adopt new coping mechanisms that do not stress your body or mind even more. If you're using substances to combat your stress, they will only intensify your stress levels. Research methods that are calming, healthy, productive, and rejuvenating.

Take five minutes to sit still and just breathe.

"The greatest weapon against stress is our ability to choose one thought over another."

—William James

UNHEARD

Have you ever sat in a room full of people and felt invisible because no one saw *you*? I mean *saw* you.

The feeling of your mouth being taped. You're screaming, but there is no sound. If you can provide something for them, you will be heard for what you can do, but not for what you have to say.

Your voice is warranted for decisions but not for discussions. You are drowned out by the noise of others' wants and needs, only to be pushed forward when you're needed.

"Are you ok?" is not a question you're familiar with, because you have learned to live in the silence of your thoughts while you're tending to everyone else.

You can't be honest, because honestly, they don't care to hear or see you. Instead, you live in the closet of your emotions and hide under the bed of your pain. You lay in the sorrows of your disappointments because no one cares to hear you.

You have learned that living on mute gets you attention, but it doesn't get you *heard* because as a little boy, you were told to MAN up and don't cry.

Mama held you to the standard of the man she never had, and now you are the man of the house with the mind of a boy who has had to function in silence by default.

You enter your world daily on silent mode, going through the motions because you were overshadowed by the women in the house who looked over your moments of silence. Now your pain is worn on your sleeve while you muster the energy to not snap at those around you.

You have locked up your thoughts and feelings and you can't find the keys because you never found your voice.

You have felt unheard all your life. Now someone is asking, "Are you ok?" They're frustrated because it's difficult for you to talk. You were never given permission to speak. They interpret your shutdown as incompetence, but the reality of your experience is that you are UNHEARD.

—King Jay

WHAT'S LOVE GOT TO DO WITH IT

So many messages encourage women to love themselves, but there are very few for men. I want to encourage you, brother, that self-LOVE is the best love you can give.

How you love on yourself will determine the love you have for others. Many times we show love by giving things, but love is an action and a choice. Dig deep, brother, in the corners of your mind and heart, and find a reason to love yourself. YOU ARE WORTHY of deep self-love.

Take time this week to begin loving on you. Take the journey of self-love because you DESERVE to experience the love you show others. Identify some things about yourself that are not external. Go deep within and explore the characteristic traits of your being. No one can ever love you better than yourself. Please don't confuse self-love with selfishness.

What does self-love mean to you?

_____

_____

_____

_____

_____

_____

_____

_____

What has kept you from loving YOU?

_____

_____

_____

_____

_____

_____

_____

_____

_____

_____

What would it feel like to be loved for who you are?

_____

_____

_____

_____

_____

_____

_____

_____

_____

Write down five ways you can begin loving on yourself. (For example: "I will begin to take time for myself before I enter the workplace as a form of self-love.")

_____

_____

_____

_____

_____

_____

_____

_____

_____

"How you love yourself is how you teach others to love you."

—Rupi Kaur

HE-EMOTIONS

Suppressing your emotions is very unhealthy. Whether you're feeling anger, grief, frustration, or sadness, they will cause your body a great deal of stress. Because your emotions aren't going away, bro, they will lie dormant until you're triggered by something or someone.

As men, most of us live on autopilot, meaning we just go through the motions. Then, one day we explode. Usually, no one saw it coming. We do a great job of hiding pain because we feel we must suppress our feelings.

Don't shut down, brother. I know you have been misunderstood feel like no one has the capacity to comfort you, and that's ok. But I want you to explore and process your deepest feelings and raw emotions this week. Take the journey of divulging your emotions and feelings with your pen.

Check in with your feelings and write about what you have been suppressing.

_____

_____

_____

_____

_____

_____

_____

_____

Connect with the emotions you feel, such as anger, sadness, or resentment.

_____

_____

_____

_____

_____

_____

_____

_____

_____

Describe in detail as best as you can what it feels like to connect with your emotions.

_____

_____

_____

_____

_____

_____

_____

_____

What emotions did you release today?

_____

_____

_____

_____

_____

_____

_____

_____

_____

"A man who is unable to connect with his emotions will remain emotionally unavailable."

—King Jay

PURPOSE

His pain stood strong chillin' in the back of the room, yet purpose had an agenda. He be that sunshine in the middle of a typhoon and didn't even know his resilience provoked his greatness.

Deep tears in his eyes as God reconstructed his heart. Purpose refused to let him fail. Covered by his mother's prayer to be better than he could ever imagine. God showed up.

Many weapons formed, but never could prosper. His eyes shifted into a newness.

Everything he touches multiples, his vision is written down, it's specific. Passionate about his purpose as he remains resilient.

God is pleased and the world is impacted, so now you see why purpose had the perfect agenda in its perfect timing.

—Written by Miss MouthPeace

DEALING WITH THE FUTURE

FEAR

The biggest misconception about fear is that being afraid isn't manly or masculine. Can I be honest with you, brother? I'm afraid more often than I would like to be. There are times I don't know if I can get the job done because I don't want to fail. Guess what? That's ok.

It's ok to be afraid. It's how you move while you're in fear that determines what will happen. It's normal and human to be afraid, but it's not ok to let the fear paralyze you to the point you do nothing.

Fear can trap us at times, and it will limit us from achieving any goal or vision we have set out to accomplish.

Fear is nothing more than an emotion that can be caused by anticipation or threat of danger. Be mindful that you do not function in the fear but outside of it. Use the fear as fuel to push you to the next step, phase, or place in your life. Acknowledging that you are afraid is self-awareness and choosing whether fear has power over you is a decision.

Take the journey of exploring your biggest fears. I challenge you to eradicate the thoughts that are keeping you from moving forward.

What is your biggest fear?

_____

_____

_____

_____

_____

_____

_____

_____

_____

What have you allowed fear to keep you from doing?

_____

_____

_____

_____

_____

_____

_____

_____

_____

If you could channel fear into fuel, what would you do?

_____

_____

_____

_____

_____

_____

_____

_____

_____

List some things that you will do outside of fear:

_____

_____

_____

_____

_____

_____

_____

_____

_____

"One of the greatest discoveries a man makes, one of his great surprises, is to find he can do what he was afraid he couldn't do."

—Henry Ford

HIGH VALUE

A re you familiar with the term "High Value?" It has become the standard most men want to achieve.

If I can, I would like to share the insight that high value doesn't equate to high functioning. Your ability to function on a high level is contingent upon the work you have done internally and not externally.

Personal achievements and high salaries are great. But are you successful in your personal life?

_____

_____

_____

_____

_____

_____

_____

_____

_____

Do you value your network or your SELF-WORK? Why?

_____

_____

_____

_____

_____

_____

_____

_____

_____

_____

What areas in life can you value more?

_____

_____

_____

_____

_____

_____

_____

_____

_____

Are you placing too much value on your exterior rather than your interior? If so, why?

_____

_____

_____

_____

_____

_____

_____

_____

Write a list of the things you value that are not tangible objects.

_____

_____

_____

_____

_____

_____

_____

_____

_____

"Every choice we make in life is a value proposition."

—Gregory Douglass

TALK TO HIM

I can remember the 13-year-old Jay. He stepped into the U-Haul truck driven by Mother on our way to Texas after my parents divorced.

I can vividly see the water in my eyes as I held onto my younger sisters. Something in me knew that life was going to change but I didn't have a clue what that would be. All I heard from other family members was that I had to be strong and be the man of the house. How, Sway? I was just a little boy who needed to be held and not thrust into this role of "man" because my father chose to walk away.

I have spent most of my life ignoring the little boy inside who was screaming for attention. Finally, when I sought therapy, I begin to speak to him occasionally and apologize for carrying so much guilt and shame, and for allowing him to experience hurt.

Brother, you can't change what happened to your younger self, but you can have a conversation. Many of us are dragging our little boy around as collateral damage and it is affecting who we can be.

Take the journey of speaking to the little boy inside you and begin to process any negative experiences or events. It was not your fault that you could not save him, but you can set the man free today.

Write a letter to the age you were when you experienced the pain that you are carrying. (Take your time and process your emotions. Do not rush the letter.) Be as raw and truthful as you can be.

_____

_____

_____

_____

_____

_____

_____

_____

_____

_____

_____

_____

_____

_____

_____

_____

_____

_____

Don't hold yourself captive because of something that happened to that little boy. It was not your fault, brother, but it's your responsibility to choose how you will move forward.

"Change the narrative by choosing you."

—King Jay

WHAT'S ON YOUR MIND?

Until you get your mind right, you'll never be able to get your life right. Why? Because nothing in your life can exceed your level of thinking. Your reality cannot supersede your mentality.

Every success or failure in life is brought about by your way of thinking. Consequently, those thoughts become the driving force of your actions. That is why so many people live a life of limitation; their life is as restricted as their thinking.

> "If you truly want to change your life, you must first change your way of thinking. Bigger and better results require a bigger and better vision for your life. So the choice is yours. You can either think your way to a whole new level or to an all-time low. Which will it be?"
>
> —Dr. John Barton

My vision is to revolutionize this nation with the Word God has placed in my belly. It is no longer a dream; it is a vision I cannot shake. I have devoted my energy, passion, and enthusiasm toward my purpose. I don't want this for fame or glory. That doesn't matter to me; all I ever wanted was to share my story of how I almost left my purpose behind. It is important to me share my story and not for glory. Glory goes to God, but it is amazing how His plan is so much better than what I anticipated. I am in constant awe because I can never predict God, but He is the greatest strategist ever. I asked God for a national stage for the opportunity to reach teens across the globe and He gave me a platform to heal men.

—King Jay

Everyone has a purpose in life and a unique talent to give to others. And when we blend this unique talent with service to others, we experience the ecstasy and exultation of own spirit, which is the ultimate goal of all goals.

—Kallam Anji Reddy

LEGACY

What will you leave behind?

Legacy. What does that word mean to you? As men, we create life through our natural function and that shouldn't be taken for granted. We have the same power Adam had when he first saw Eve and called her WOMAN.

Adam named all the animals in the kingdom because God granted him authority over whatever he spoke (manifested).

As you're working through this journal and writing your thoughts and feelings, think about what you will create with your words. What will you leave behind?

What will the legacy of your last name be? How will you be remembered on the day your funeral? I know that is a rather challenging question, but I want you to go there, brother, and begin processing the word *legacy*.

It is my mission to leave a legacy of healing and building people to become the best version of themselves through addressing unresolved trauma. I want my future family to know their father worked his purpose so they could live their purpose.

I want to leave a legacy of functioning and healthy behaviors, not perfection but self-awareness and the ability to pivot when life happens.

It's not about how you are remembered but rather the memories of your existence that will hold weight in the hearts and minds of those who will come behind you.

Take the journey this week to think about your legacy and the memory you wish for others to hold in their minds about you.

"Legacy is not what I did for myself. It's what I'm doing for the next generation."
—Vitor Belfort

What does legacy mean to you?

_____

_____

_____

_____

_____

_____

_____

_____

_____

_____

_____

How do you want people to remember you?

_____

_____

_____

_____

_____

_____

_____

_____

_____

What are some things you can do to begin working on your legacy?

_____

_____

_____

_____

_____

_____

_____

_____

What do you want to leave behind for the next generation?

_____

_____

_____

_____

_____

_____

_____

What life lessons would you give to a young man to encourage him?

_____

_____

_____

_____

_____

_____

_____

_____

"Your legacy is the summation of the life you lead, not the life you posted."

—King Jay

WHAT IS A MAN?

Dear brother,

As I've pondered the question, "What exactly is a man?" I discovered a deeply rooted question that was buried within me. How do I become this man I've never witnessed? Pondering through society's wide scope had me lost within the very scales of my own life. How can I identify with someone who broke me at birth? An absent man!

Born into that (fatherless) plague created a rollercoaster filled with the failures of unbalanced emotions. I assumed that being intimate with women would validate this man I was searching for. Body after body, void still unmet.

Crazy, I didn't realize I was becoming angrier and more numb after each failed attempt. Why? Since my dad wasn't there, I tried to be validated by whatever I touched. One day God told me to look in the mirror. All I could see was pain. I began to weep profusely, head bent.

I heard God say, "Lift your head and face your pain."

Man, that was tough, facing my demons, and dealing with the ugly I created within myself while blaming others for my actions.

That was the first time I took responsibility! People often say, "man up," but if you have never seen a man who is up, those words are foreign. God showed me I was a man who had to get up. I am the blueprint. What I've been looking for was always planted within me. But I had to stop blaming everyone and hold myself accountable.

I then discovered what a man is. A man is human. A man is spiritual. A man can cry. A man can be vulnerable. A man can have emotions that even he does not understand. A man can take a blank canvas with no identity and give it life. A man can heal and love.

How do I know this? Because I became the man I never knew how to be. That man is me. I have been defined by God's strength. It wasn't about people believing in me. It was about me believing in who God created me to be and accepting everything about me, no matter who was or wasn't there, no matter who agrees with me or not. I became unapologetically me! A man who inspires many to live. A man many look to as a brother, a father, a son, and a friend.

Guess what? There was no blueprint to becoming this man. The key was not to feel sorry for myself and invite you on my journey. So, what is a man? A man is you, and the brothers who chose not to just survive but thrive. They understand divine assignment and make a promise to pass the baton of excellence down to the next generation of Kings! Together we break generational curses. I am my brother's keeper!

—Shareeff A. Delacruz

BE HEALED

In Webster's dictionary, the word "Heal" means to make free from injury or disease. I rather like the latter meaning, which is to make sound or WHOLE.

Healing is about undoing the effects of what was done so we can move from surviving to thriving.

We have carried our hurt far too long, bro. It's time to break free from the traumas of the past and the pain of its memory.

Our families are depending on us to lead them to better lives through our example of living, not with our accomplishments or money. So many people want to build generational wealth, but true wealth begins with healing.

We have seen enough of generational dysfunctions and unhealed behaviors. It's time to change that for the next generation.

Let's pass down healthy communication skills, healthy boundaries, and positive thinking that serve us well.

Use this time and journal to start the process of your healing. Healing looks different for everyone, so remain focused on your path to freedom.

Cry when you need to, scream, tear up some paper, or go for a run. Find a way, bro, to fight your way out. Don't allow the enemy to steal what is rightfully yours: FREEDOM.

You have a right to heal and a right to be free. But it won't be easy, and only you can do the work.

Don't throw in the towel, brother. Your life means something to those around you, whether you believe it or not.

Hold on, brother. Help is here.

This journal is nothing more than a tool such as prayer, in which you talk to the source of your belief. The difference is that you are talking from within by writing your thoughts. The more you journal, the more liberating it becomes.

Lean into the healing space to release the burden you have been carrying all these years. Set the little boy free, so the man can live without restraint and limitation.

What has kept you from pursuing your healing?

_____

_____

_____

_____

_____

_____

_____

_____

_____

_____

How important is healing to you?

_____

_____

_____

_____

_____

_____

_____

_____

_____

How can you continue your healing process?

_____

_____

_____

_____

_____

_____

_____

_____

_____

What are some things you will begin healing?

_____

_____

_____

_____

_____

_____

_____

_____

How will healing improve your life?

_____

_____

_____

_____

_____

_____

_____

_____

As I close out this journal, continue to do the work daily because HEALING IS A JOURNEY and WHOLENESS is the destination.

Just Heal, Bro

Daily Thoughts

Daily Thoughts

Daily Thoughts

Daily Thoughts

_____

_____

_____

_____

_____

_____

_____

_____

_____

_____

_____

_____

_____

_____

_____

_____

_____

_____

_____

_____

_____

_____

Daily Thoughts

Daily Thoughts

_____

_____

_____

_____

_____

_____

_____

_____

_____

_____

_____

_____

_____

_____

_____

_____

_____

_____

_____

_____

_____

Made in the USA
Columbia, SC
03 April 2025

56106598R00057